Stop Lusting
&
Start Living

A Sexual Battle
and
Recovery Plan

By

Paul F. Davis

"Follow peace with all men, and holiness, without which no man shall see the Lord: Looking diligently lest any man fail of the grace of God; lest any root of bitterness springing up trouble you, and thereby many be defiled; Lest there be any fornicator, or profane person, as Esau, who for one morsel of meat sold his birthright. For you know how that afterward, when he would have inherited the blessing, he was rejected: for he found no place of repentance, though he sought it carefully with tears" (Hebrews 12:14-17).

"Let us hear the conclusion of the whole matter: Fear God, and keep His commandments: for this is the whole duty of man. For God shall bring every work into judgment, with every secret thing, whether it be good, or whether it be evil" (Ecclesiastes 12:13-14).

Introduction

This book is a battle plan and strategy for sexual recovery, wherein I transparently share my personal experiences as a young man after having given my life to God. I have not edited this book much from the time it was originally written. It details many of my battles trying to remain pure unto God and faithful to my wife when I was married.

As you know the Word of God and truth is timeless, tested and endures for all generations. So too shall the Spirit of God, which moves in wisdom, power and love; comfort every person in need of the blessings found in this book and others I have written that strengthen one's manhood and individual core at the center of every human being.

Among the blessings to be found herein are inner healing (read my book "Breakthrough For A Broken Heart" for more on this topic too), a renewed identity (read my book "Update Your Identity" to fully grasp and understand why this is important if you hunger for more at the end of this book), and divine restoration to settle, establish and lift you up to where you belong so you can live free, be happy and have a grounded inner focus to direct your life and fulfill your higher purpose for which you were created by God.

As for me and my story when I was most fiercely wrestling with trying to control my physical body; I quickly learned this battle requires spiritual weapons, divine truth, and supernatural power to win it.

Upon continually being carried away repeatedly by my own lusts (while yet single, working as a lifeguard at a Central Florida water park and preparing to attend Bible College to be trained to enter the ministry - long before I was ever married), I began crying out to God to "deliver me from evil." I said to God, "Deliver me and I will deliver others." The Lord replied, "You shall deliver nations." For this reason my insights are being put in print to deliver the peoples of the earth from diverse lusts and a wayward life.

Deliverance comes in many forms and fashions. For myself Providence has seemingly had deliverance to come to me through the gaining of personal revelatory insight in regard to sexuality and the forces thereof. This book therefore has written me as much as I have written it. My fingers are the pen of a ready writer within, that being the Spirit of the Lord (Psalm 45:1).

God's Word declares: "through knowledge shall the just be delivered" (Proverbs 11:9 b). Three types of knowledge are instrumental for succeeding in any endeavor, sex included. They are the knowledge of oneself, the knowledge others, and the knowledge of God. Personal transformation in regard to one's sexuality cannot occur apart from a discovery of oneself and a discovery of the divine Creator. Self discovery demands that a personal inventory be conducted – often times a process too painful for many people to endure.

Upon awaking one morning and feeling condemned for my continual struggle against my flesh throughout the week, the Lord said: "You need a sex plan." I always try to read God's Word first thing in the morning and take some time to pray before beginning my day. It is quite common for me to hear God speak to me in an intimate way. Yet this was a first as to the timing and content of what God was speaking to me. Even now I am still discovering and endeavoring to fully develop this "sex plan" where I can be both prudent and premeditate my determined course of action so as to be pleasing to God and abide in my heavenly calling.

Nobody said it was going to be easy. Christianity is a strong man's religion. As for the prescription, I'm reminded that most medicines don't taste good going down. Nevertheless, if endured they can often be precisely just what is needed to facilitate the cure. It is my hope that this sexual recovery plan will be that both for you the reader and me the writer.

As it is a plan, it necessitates adherence in order to procure results. The just rightly use the God given knowledge in their possession. This sexual recovery plan is intertwined with Biblical knowledge. Any misuse or lack of use of this plan therefore on our part after having read, related to, and identified with it would be *unjust* unless we were powerless to obey it.

It is my belief that we are in fact just that – powerless – apart from the help of a loving and mighty God. Perhaps this is why so many sincere people with good intentions to bridle and harness uncontrollable lust have miserably failed. The flesh is an element that is not easily tamed without the help of the human spirit and the empowerment of the Holy Spirit.

It is for this reason that spiritual truths will be taught in this book. Only through the Spirit can we consistently and competently crucify the lusts of the body (Romans 8:13). Our bodily appetites daily war against our soul and seek to bring us into captivity. To solely surrender our souls to gratify our fleshly lusts is to reckon our minds carnal and incompetent for all other purposes.

"To be carnally minded is death; but to be spiritually minded is life and peace" (Romans 8:6). Death is not merely physical. Death can occur within when we are continually inwardly fixated on sex and gratifying our bodily appetites to the extent and expense of repressing what is really important in life. Unreasonable demands on our time and energy to feed our insatiable fleshly lusts endanger our ability to focus on our work, maintain meaningful relationships, and manage our finances. Such losses brought on by overwhelming and uncontrollable fleshly demands could definitely work havoc in our inner life and cause a slow death within the human soul.

Everyone's personal sexual recovery plan will be peculiar to their particular set of temptations. Everybody has different buttons and variables that are capable of throwing them into compulsive behavior. It is up to you therefore to ultimately pinpoint your own peculiar temptations and design a plan with your deliverance in mind. Let my plan however develop a desire for *sexual sobriety* within you and provoke you toward self-discovery and recovery.

Jesus understands better than anyone else what it is like to undergo physical temptation. God chose to dwell on earth in a man's body rather than a woman's. Therefore Christ being both God and man knew full well what it was like to deal with rapid-fire sexual desire. In all points like we, He was tempted (Hebrews 2:18; 4:15). Yet He continually submitted His will to the will of the Father so as to be perfected and thereby be able to sanctify all who would believe in His name (Matthew 26:39,42).

The key is to crucify our selfish lusts and set our affections on the risen Christ (Colossians 3:1-3).

Stop Lusting and Start Living

1. Sexual Revolution

2. Understanding the Body

3. Self Control

4. Relating to the Opposite Sex and Sin

5. Destroying Delilah and Jezebel

6. Deliverance from Demonic Influences

7. The Sword of the Lord

8. Mended for Marriage

1. Sexual Revolution

Forms of sexual expression have progressed and become increasingly blatant over the past few decades. Since the creation of television our society has been increasingly capable of viewing images affecting sexuality. It used to be a big deal for Hollywood to show women's shoulders, belly button, or a dress above the knees. Today, we have far surpassed that and are pushing each generation's level of tolerance further toward complete nudity. The hippie days of the Woodstock era, in which everyone said "Peace" and "Love," opened the door to promiscuity and "free sex" void of any marital commitment.

As I writer I seek to relate rather than to Pontificate. Research and reason is sufficient to enable anyone to recognize that we have a real problem with our sexuality. Unsettled in our sexuality, our individual identity remains unstable and therefore our behavior problematic.

Many of us have common characteristics in regard to our sexuality. Realizing that you are not alone in your struggle for sexual purity is a big relief as you seek to sort yourself out sexually.

Sexual Compulsives Anonymous lists fourteen characteristics many of us seem to have in common.

1. As adolescents, we used fantasy and compulsive masturbation to avoid feelings, and continued this tendency into our adult lives with compulsive sex.

2. Compulsive sex became a drug, which we used to escape from feelings such as anxiety, loneliness, anger and self-hatred, as well as joy.

3. We tended to become immobilized by romantic obsessions. We became addicted to the search for sex and

love; as a result, we neglected our lives.

4. We sought oblivion in fantasy and masturbation, and lost ourselves in compulsive sex. Sex became a reward, punishment, distraction and time-killer.

5. Because of our low self-esteem, we used sex to feel validated and complete.

6. We tried to bring intensity and excitement into our lives through sex, but felt ourselves growing steadily emptier.

7. Sex was compartmentalized instead of integrated into our lives as a healthy element.

8. We became addicted to people, and were unable to distinguish among sex, love and affection.

9. We searched for some "magical" quality in others to make us feel complete. Other people were idealized and endowed with a powerful symbolism, which often disappeared after we had sex with them.

10. We were drawn to people who were not available to us, or who would reject or abuse us.

11. We feared relationships, but continually searched for them. In a relationship, we feared abandonment

and rejection, but out of one, we felt empty and incomplete.

12. While constantly seeking intimacy with another person, we found that the desperate quality of our need made true intimacy with anyone impossible, and we often developed unhealthy dependency relationships that eventually became unbearable.

13. Even when we got the love of another person, it never seemed enough, and we were unable to stop lusting after others.

14. Trying to conceal our dependency demands, we grew more isolated from ourselves, from God, and from the very people we longed to be

close to. (http://www.sca-recovery.org/Characteristics.html, 1996)

The first common characteristic, the avoidance of feelings, is worth investigating and deciphering. Feelings are a funny thing because they are continually given to change. In fact feelings are much like roller coasters. They quickly go up and they go down. The rapidity with which our feelings fluctuate can be quite mind-boggling. Particularly men, who are typically less in touch with their feelings than women, find females at times to be quite moody.

Regardless of our gender, feelings are something we all must learn to deal with and properly handle. An improper handling of our feelings can further frustrate and aggravate the problem that brought on the negative feelings to begin with. We therefore must strive to locate the root of the feelings that most torment us and cause us to experience discomfort.

Avoidance of feelings that we dislike or perhaps don't know how to explain, can lead us into wrongful habits that are destructive and break us down. There used to be a commercial for stomach disorders, which said, "How do you spell relief?" That is an important question we all must ask ourselves. Because *the way we rid ourselves of painful emotions and disheartening feelings will either further take us deeper into bondage or assure our continuous liberty.*

Many have chosen to simply avoid and not deal with negative feelings, in hopes that they will one day just go away. Such people often find that what they use to spell "relief" eventually becomes like a drug to them. For many that drug is sex. When a person reaches such a point where their relief mechanism (be it here sex) used to rid their inner agony becomes an addiction, they go from sex being a complimentary component within their life to a compulsion that enslaves and drives them.

Immobilization and personal neglect is the norm for many starving for love and affection. Upon reaching the depths of personal neglect, many people are truly not capable of genuine relational intimacy until they themselves are first restored individually. Not until one's inner self is healed and restored can true intimacy be established with others.

Inner healing cannot come unless you are first willing to be brutally honest with yourself and acknowledge your unhealthy dependencies. Most people choose not to acknowledge their inner needs and ask for help. Instead they conceal their need for dependency and isolate themselves, which serves to further intensify the problem.

Self-assessment and acknowledging our problems in life is vitally important to ensure personal well-being. Sex Addicts Anonymous has a useful tool for self-assessment in the 12 Questions they ask to assess sexual addiction in a person. They are as follows:

1. Do you keep secrets about your sexual or romantic activities from those important to you? Do you lead a double life?

2. Have your needs driven you to have sex in places or situations or with

people you would not normally choose?

3. Do you find yourself looking for sexually arousing articles or scenes in newspapers, magazines, or other media?

4. Do you find that romantic or sexual fantasies interfere with your relationships or are preventing you from facing problems?

5. Do you frequently want to get away from a sex partner after having sex? Do you frequently feel remorse, shame, or guilt after a sexual encounter?

6. Do you feel shame about your body or your sexuality, such that you avoid touching your body or engaging in sexual relationships? Do you fear that you have no sexual feelings, that you are asexual?

7. Does each new relationship continue to have the same destructive patterns, which prompted you to leave the last relationship?

8. Is it taking more variety and frequency of sexual and romantic activities than previously to bring the same levels of excitement and relief?

9. Have you ever been arrested or are you in danger of being arrested because of your practices of

voyeurism, exhibitionism, prostitution, sex with minors, indecent phone calls, etc.?

10. Does your pursuit of sex or romantic relationships interfere with your spiritual beliefs or development?

11. Do your sexual activities include the risk, threat, or reality of disease, pregnancy, coercion, or violence?

12. Has your sexual or romantic behavior ever left you feeling hopeless, alienated from others, or suicidal?

I remember when I was in high school, guys in the locker room would boast about which girl they had been with and how they had performed. The conversation, jokes, and attitudes toward the opposite sex that I came in contact with gradually began to affect me. Eventually, I too was giving over my ears and mind to the topic of sex. Upon giving myself to engage in sexual activity at the premarital level, I found myself somewhat disoriented during the act and socially dysfunctional afterward. I was speechless both because of the immense fleshly gratification and the inability to appropriately communicate with the girl with whom I had participated in intercourse.

Basically, I was physically mature enough to perform the act of sex but inwardly and soulishly inept at providing any emotional comfort to she with whom I had been sexually engaged. Honestly I just wanted to leave after having intercourse, as I felt quite awkward. Furthermore after having been personally gratified, I saw no further reason to remain with the young lady and left to go play ball. Undoubtedly this had lust written all over it and love was nowhere to be found.

It behooves us to ask the right questions before engaging in sex so that we can avoid this feeling of awkwardness once we enter the bedchamber. Perhaps answering some simple questions will provide us some foresight and insight that merely hindsight (after the fact) cannot give us.

Let us look at the "Twenty Questions" asked by Sexual Compulsives Anonymous (http://www.sca-recovery.org/Questions.html).

1. Do you frequently experience remorse, depression, or guilt about your sexual activity?

2. Do you feel your sexual drive and activity is getting out of control? Have you repeatedly tried to stop or reduce certain sexual behaviors, but inevitably you could not?

3. Are you unable to resist sexual advances, or turn down sexual propositions when offered?

4. Do you use sex to escape from uncomfortable feelings such as anxiety, fear, anger, resentment, guilt, etc. which seem to disappear when the sexual obsession starts?

5. Do you spend excessive time obsessing about sex or engaged in sexual activity?

6. Have you neglected your family, friends, spouse or relationship because of the time you spend in sexual activity?

7. Do your sexual pursuits interfere with your work or professional development?

8. Is your sexual life secretive, a source of shame, and not in keeping with

your values? Do you lie to others to cover up your sexual activity?

9. Are you afraid of sex? Do you avoid romantic and sexual relationships with others and restrict your sexual activity to fantasy, masturbation, and solitary or anonymous activity?

10. Are you increasingly unable to perform sexually without other stimuli such as pornography, videos, "poppers," drugs/alcohol, "toys," etc.?

11. Do you have to resort increasingly to abusive, humiliating, or painful sexual fantasies or behaviors to get sexually aroused?

12. Has your sexual activity prevented you from developing a close, loving relationship with a partner? Or, have you developed a pattern of intense romantic or sexual relationships that never seem to last once the excitement wears off?

13. Do you only have anonymous sex or one-night stands? Do you usually want to get away from your sexual partner after the encounter?

14. Do you have sex with people with whom you normally would not associate?

15. Do you frequent clubs, bars, adult bookstores, restrooms, parks and

other public places in search of sexual partners?

16. Have you ever been arrested or placed yourself in legal jeopardy for your sexual activity?

17. Have you ever risked your physical health with exposure to sexually transmitted diseases, especially AIDS, by engaging in "unsafe" sexual activity?

18. Has the money you spent on pornography, videos, phone sex, or hustlers/prostitutes strained your financial resources?

19. Have people you trust expressed concern about your sexual activity?

20. Does life seem meaningless and
hopeless without a romantic or
sexual relationship?

The sex drive touches every component of the person. For that reason the sex drive must be handled with care and respect. If abused or allowed to have its own way, the sex drive can destroy you completely. The sex drive can debilitate your body and corrupt your soul, while alienating your spirit. Our handling of the sex drive is therefore a very serious matter.

Sex has become the most discussed but least understood aspect of human life. Sexual intercourse is an act, which affects the whole personality. Intercourse is a personal encounter between a man and a woman in the depths of their being, which does something permanent to each, for good, or for ill.

Looking back in retrospect, my first sexual experience (premarital, during my B.C. days) was as if my flesh had reached the peak of arousal and my soul had collapsed within to the Grand Canyon. This is quite surprising as I was not practicing any religion at the time, nor was I devout in any way. Mentally I felt no guilt whatsoever, though the thought of pregnancy did come to mind as I in my youthful zeal had neglected to consider the possibility of conception. The state of my soul following sexual intercourse affirms to me (now looking back in retrospect) that sex apart from a marital commitment is destructive to the souls of the individuals engaged.

Despite the excessive boasting of our sexual exploits, we are living in the Sexual Dark Ages. *Though we hear more about sex than our parents or grandparents ever heard, we understand much less.* It is not uncommon for many people in society to talk sex, see sex, think and dream sex, but yet be totally ignorant of God's purpose for sex.

We have a whole new entourage of helping professionals that try to untangle the knot of confused sexual mores, while profiting handsomely in the meantime. Many people's sexual orbit is continually changing according to the dictates of Hollywood and the latest sexually driven song on MTV.

Yet without a divine understanding of sex and a realization that God created us to be sexual creatures, sex can become confusing and agonizing. Our generation has played with the sex drive as if it were a toy. We've sought immediate gratification at the expense of personal fulfillment. Fleeting sexual fun has left us inwardly empty and seeking for more, never to be fulfilled.

Nearly every book of the Bible mentions sex directly or indirectly. God has given us in His Word some very direct, explicit commands regarding sex. If we keep His commands, we shall enjoy sex as it is to be enjoyed. If we however defy His laws, we shall bring suffering upon ourselves.

Suffering can be avoided as we discipline ourselves to keep God's commandments despite our feelings and thoughts. Sexual purity has been said to be achieved when you are not gratified by anything or anyone other than your spouse. Of course if you're not married, gratification should come primarily from your Creator and the joys of life itself beyond the bedroom.

Sexual Revolution – prophetic principles

God doesn't want us sinning against our own bodies. The wages of sin is death (Romans 6:23).

There is nothing wrong with struggling. It's when we quit struggling and give in that there is a problem.

Everyone's personal sexual recovery plan will be peculiar to their particular set of temptations.

Develop a desire for sexual sobriety.

Be established in your identity, settled in your sexuality and disciplined behaviorally.

Feelings are funny because they are continually given to change.

An improper handling of our feelings can further frustrate and aggravate the problem that brought on the negative feelings to begin with.

The way we rid ourselves of painful emotions and disheartening feelings will either further take us deeper into bondage or assure our continuous liberty.

Immobilization and personal neglect is the norm for many starving for love and affection.

It is best to be restored inwardly before seeking relationship outwardly. Nevertheless both often can occur simultaneously.

God has given us in His Word some very direct, explicit commands regarding sex.

2. Understanding the Body

Understanding the body in its proper place and context is paramount in order to live in harmony with yourself. The God of peace wants to "sanctify you wholly" and preserve your whole spirit, soul, and body blameless unto the coming of our Lord Jesus Christ (1 Thes. 5:23). If God is going to great lengths to try to preserve our spirit, soul, and body; then conversely something and someone is seeking to devour our spirit, soul, and body.

Keep in mind you are a spirit. You have a mind. And you live in a body. Contrary to popular belief, your body is NOT you. If I put my hand in a baseball glove and move it, the life is not in the glove. The source of life and movement is the hand within the glove. The human body is no different. The body without the spirit is dead (James 2:26).

A human being apart from God is dead in trespasses and sins (Eph.2:1-2). His conversation and pursuits being fleshly continually reveal this. Overtaken by the desires of the flesh and carnal mind, he is a child of wrath destined for eternal separation and damnation. Though a child of wrath, on earth he is a lover of the world. He is fully given over to the lust of the flesh, the lust of the eyes, and the pride of life (1 Jn.2:16). Yet the world and all its lusts pass away, but he that does the will of God will abide forever (v. 17).

Overcome by his own lusts, he is a servant of corruption (2 Pet.2:19). Brought into bondage by his own lusts and ultimately overcome, he is unable to harness himself. Like an ox going to the slaughter, the man governed solely by his flesh will soon come to his own ruin. Furthermore the body without the spirit "genders to bondage" (or is inclined to bondage and decay) as the beauty thereof fades away (Gal.4:23-24).

Beauty is vain (Proverbs 31:30). "All flesh is grass, and all the goodliness thereof is as the flower of the field: The grass withers, the flower fades: because the spirit of the Lord blows upon it: surely the people is grass" (Isaiah 40:6-7).

Sex is a God Idea

Sex is God's idea and therefore is good. It is best however within the perimeters of a marital relationship. Sex should be used, but in its proper place and time, according to God's plan. Outside of God's plan, it quickly becomes a means of division, a source of cruelty, perversion, and death.

The Bible talks honestly about the human sex drive. In fact, it is more forthright and honest in describing the sex drive than many of the so-called sex manuals published. Take a look at Judges 14:1-2. This passage describes how a young Israelite named Samson visited the Philistine territory of Timnath. Notice what happened when Samson went back home. As soon as he met his mother and father, he said, "I have seen a woman in Timnath of the daughters of the Philistines: now therefore get her for me to wife" (v.2). Here a young man sees an attractive woman and on first impulse he says, "I want her!"

Better than love at first sight is love with divine insight. Samson's life depicts this truth, as he had to lose his eyesight before he could regain his insight. Samson found himself in the lap of the woman of his dreams only to be devastated and destroyed by her (Judg.16). Indeed, a guy who falls in love with a girl at first sight often wishes he had taken a second look.

One woman was asked why she was wearing her wedding ring on the wrong finger. She replied, "It's because I married the wrong man." Nowadays couples have the honeymoon first: If it's a success, they have the engagement, and if that works out all right, they may have a wedding.

When Adam was lonely, God created for him one wife, not ten friends. Furthermore, God created Adam and Eve, not Adam and Steve. Nowadays animals have more sense than many humans when it comes to sex. Our generation is full of people who are bisexual, transsexual and homosexual. In actuality these perversions repress their true sexuality and make them asexual. This explains why so many engaged in strange sexual lifestyles feel the need to verbally assert their sexuality, because within their heart they honestly cannot confidently validate their sexuality. Their self image is distorted and thus they are seeking to be validated and accepted.

Sex has become the most discussed but least understood aspect of human life. The extent to which magazines, talk shows, and books discuss the topic of sex leaves humans in a mad frenzy to apprehend all the information they possibly can as sex is erroneously portrayed as the ultimate in life itself.

I certainly would not argue sex is not highly enjoyable, neither would I seek to remove the place sex holds in a marital relationship. Yet the obsessive manner in which people pursue and discuss the topic is abnormal. Could it be they who talk the most about sex experience it the least? Perhaps all the big mouth sex doctors are like the perennial youth at school who boasts to his friends about the sexual exploits he never had.

No matter who you are, no matter what your background is, something inside you draws you to the opposite sex. God made you that way. All of His creation is interrelated. God created males and females to be attracted to one another. God gave each person an endowment of physical forces – "drives". The sex drive is not evil and therefore should not be ignored. It must be understood and controlled.

What is evil is when you allow your body to take over the affairs of your life and essentially rule you. God intended for you by the strength of the spirit within to govern your flesh. Those who are governed by their bodily appetites find themselves becoming increasingly vile as they venture into more odd sex acts and unbecoming behavior to satisfy their insatiable lust. The apostle Paul gives us some understanding concerning the human body when he calls his flesh, "my vile body" (Phil.3:21). Paul said, "I know that in me [that is, in my flesh] dwells no good thing" (Rom. 7:18).

Understanding that the extent to which you rule your body will determine your state of mental health, you should exercise all due care to examine and harness your fleshly lusts. What you do with your body affects your mind.

"For this is the will of God, even your sanctification, that you should abstain from fornication: That every one of you should KNOW HOW to possess his vessel [body] in sanctification and honor." (I Thes.4:3-4)

Many of us know WHAT we should be doing, but do not KNOW HOW. The will is present, but HOW TO PERFORM we don't know (Romans 7:18).

As we progress onward in our pursuit and discussion of the abundant life in Christ, we shall herein give practical ways that will tell us *how to perform* that which is godly and right.

Understanding the Body – prophetic principles

Your body is NOT you!

A human being apart from God is dead in trespasses and sins (Eph.2:1-2).

The world and all its lusts pass away, but he that does the will of God will abide forever (1 John 2:17).

Like an ox going to the slaughter, the man governed solely by his flesh will soon come to his own ruin.

Sex is God's idea and therefore is good. It is best however within the perimeters of a marital relationship.

Outside of God's plan sex quickly becomes a means of division, a source of cruelty, perversion, and death.

When we keep our body in check and its rightful place, our life remains balanced. Our body must be kept in its proper place otherwise it will get out of line and think to control you. It is you who are to control your body.

Better than love at first sight is love with insight.

A woman who falls in love with a man at first sight often wishes she had taken a second look.

One woman was asked why she was wearing her wedding ring on the wrong finger. She replied, "It's because I married the wrong man."

No matter how spiritual you become your body will still cry for food, sleep, and sex. You may be sanctified, but your flesh wants to be satisfied.

When Adam was lonely, God created for him one wife, not ten friends.

Men's eyes are like lasers that intensely zoom in on female flesh. Men are visually stimulated through their eyes.

Women are stimulated audibly. It's the ears of a woman that are never satisfied. That's why they are so easily given to gossip.

What you do with your body effects your mind.

Impulsive people tend to act on a moment's notice when an impulse or urge excites them. Such sudden and spontaneous inclinations to perform an unpremeditated action can be destructive if the impelling force is the flesh.

Sex has become the most discussed but least understood aspect of human life.

3. Self Control

Self-control is the exercise of restraint over one's own impulses, emotions, and desires. Impulsive people tend to act on a moment's notice when an impulse or urge excites them. Such sudden and spontaneous inclinations to perform an unpremeditated action can be destructive if the impelling force is the flesh.

Impulses transmitted by the Spirit of God however can be quite good and serve to bless our lives. The fruit of God's Spirit is love, joy, peace, patience, kindness, gentleness, and self-control (Galatians 5:22-23).

It behooves us to evaluate and examine our urges to see whether they are of the flesh or the Spirit. Stimulation unaccounted for and blindly followed can be extremely dangerous. Merely going by feeling can be harmful. A frog can give you a feeling and then urinate on you.

Allow me to give a crude illustration I once heard a young lady give from a youth group I formerly attended. She said, "Sin is like poop on a beautiful silver platter. It's covered with chocolate syrup, whip-cream, nuts and dressed all up. Then you begin to eat and it seemingly tastes good. Then all of the sudden you get to the center and discover you've been eating dung. Of course, you're immediately disgusted and sick within. That is how sin is."

The media and TV make sexual promiscuity outside of marriage appear fun and permissible. God however says, "Flee fornication. Every sin that a man does is without the body, but he that commits fornication sins against his own body" (1Corinthians 6:18).

Scripture exhorts us to "Flee youthful lusts" (II Timothy 2:22). Some would question God and say "Why?" Never put a question mark where God has put a period. No wed, no bed. If you're getting hot and bothered take a cold shower, go to the gym, call a brother in the Lord who you can pray with.

God doesn't want us sinning against our own bodies. The wages of sin is death (Romans 6:23). This is why many get sexually transmitted diseases, prostate cancer, and cervical cancer. It's God's judgment and punishment for disobeying His commandments. Jesus said, "Sin no more, lest a worse thing comes upon you" (John 5:14). To avoid fornication God lets every man have his own wife.

Among the cravings of the flesh are – food, sleep, and sex. Life without an awakened spirit is purposeless and self-centered. It is for this reason we are encouraged to "bring it [the body] into subjection" (I Corinth.9:27). When we keep our body in check and its rightful place, our life remains balanced. Our body must be kept in its proper place otherwise it will get out of line and think to control you. It is you who are to control your body.

No matter how spiritual you become your body will still cry for food, sleep, and sex. You may be sanctified, but your flesh wants to be satisfied. Thankfully, God gives grace and glory (Ps.84:11). No good thing will God withhold from them that walk uprightly. Wait on the Lord and He will do it. He will satisfy you by His Spirit and enable you to victoriously put to death the lusts of the flesh (Rom.8:13). Furthermore, our God will bless you in the fullness of time by bringing you into a perfect marital union with the person of His choosing for your life.

Meanwhile, your eyes must be single. Jesus said, "The light of the body is the eye: if therefore your eye be single, your whole body shall be full of light. But if your eye be evil, your whole body shall be full of darkness" (Matthew 6:22-23). Jesus warns that "whosoever looks on a woman to lust after her has committed adultery with her already in his heart" (Matt.5:28). Beware of optical adultery.

Make a covenant with your eyes (Job 31:1). Know what God has portioned and allotted to you. (Job 31:2) Be content therewith. Godliness with contentment is great gain (1 Tim.6:6).

Men's eyes are like lasers that intensely zoom in on female flesh. Men are visually stimulated through their eyes. That is the way God constructed us, to be visually stimulated. The danger in that is when we open ourselves up to lustful behavior and begin to visually check women out all the time as if it were a sport, or as if we were hunting for game.

"Hell and destruction are never full; so the eyes of a man are never satisfied" (Prov.27:20). Lift up your eyes, look up and think on that which is above (Jn.4:35; Prov.15:24). Looking to the left and the right will only take you to hell beneath.

Notice Jesus did not mention the eyes of a woman. Women are stimulated audibly. It's the ears of a woman that are never satisfied. Women like to hear niceties and pleasantries. One song says, "Killing me softly with his whisper and words…"

Fixating your eyes on someone transmits mental images which are then burned in the brain and become hard to get rid of. What you continually look at gets bigger. What we continually behold, good or bad, we are compelled to become. This is why the Bible exhorts us to behold the glory of the Lord, that we can be changed from glory to glory (2Cor.3:18).

There are many tempting parking spots on the road to success. We therefore must learn to bounce our eyes! When we starve our eyes from feasting on females, we further increase our spiritual hunger and godly strength within. Feed the spirit and starve the flesh.

Don't Waste Your Mind

A mind is a terrible thing to waste, misuse and neglect. For us to be whole in our soul, we must strive to fully develop our mind. The mind houses your attitudes, thoughts, and mental images. The mind generates and produces mental images according to the thoughts, concepts and ideas you give it to work with. God in His

Word declares that He sees our inner thoughts and imagery (Ezekiel 8:12).

God will render unto us the fruit of our thoughts (Jeremiah 6:19). We therefore must be extremely careful what we allow to circulate and camp out in our minds. Thoughts produce images. Images lead to actions; actions form habits; habits lead to strongholds. (II Corinth.10:3-6)

Sexual fantasies within the movie screen of your mind can be very deceiving and destructive. It can become so real that what occurs within your mind means more to you than your very own real life. Many men in marital relationships with the wife that God gave them for ultimate fulfillment and satisfaction find themselves relationally impotent due to mental fantasia keeping them involved elsewhere.

Mental fantasies lead to phony sex acts, wherewith you fantasize of the person you want to be with and in the movie screen of your mind perform the act. Such mental masturbation eventually manifests in physical masturbation. Yet there is no comparison to the real thing. Masturbation is not God's plan for man. It is essentially like playing tennis by yourself, not so fun. Get real and get a life!

When a person masturbates they set up that image in their mind as an idol and bow down to it. When someone masturbates they bring themselves into bondage because the more they give into it, the more stimuli they need to arouse themselves the next time. The result is they continue to dive deeper into the sewer of sin and bondage. (Genesis 38:9-10; 1Corinthians 6:12)

Excessive mental fantasizing can result in a wet dream. Scripture does not condemn one who has a nocturnal emission as this physical occurrence can also be the result of a build up of male testosterone that needs to be naturally released (Leviticus 15:1-10). However don't go fantasizing in your mind looking for a pleasurable dream to fill your senses. Mental masturbation can be highly destructive.

Present your body to God as a living sacrifice and be renewed in the spirit of your mind. It's your responsibility to control your body and mind. (Romans 12:1-2) Work out your salvation from the spirit man so it affects and thereby rules and governs your mind and flesh. (Philippians 2:12-13) Make your body a slave to righteousness (Romans 6:16).

Attitudes of the Heart

Beware of roots of bitterness which the devil would seek to sow in your heart in an attempt to get you to justify wrongdoing on your part. Strife opens the door to every evil work in your life. (James 3:16) Offenses cause your heart to grow hard and become incapable of hearing from God.

Life affords us ample opportunity to be offended with people, but love enables us to endure all things.

Often when you put unrealistic expectations on a person and they disappoint you, the devil will send a lying spirit to begin to tell you your rights. *You can be dead right* as far as the world is concerned *but dead wrong* and committing sin as God sees it.

Self control is exercised more easily when you have built a strong inner man through prayer and reading of God's Word (Ephesians 3:16). Joseph had a strong inner man and therefore ran from Potiphar's wife. Samson on the other hand, sat in the lap of Delilah.

Accountability Precedes Recovery

Remain accountable to men who can ask you: "How's your eyes?" "Are you successfully bringing under your bodily appetites? Are you struggling particularly with anything that I can pray about?"

Statistics show that 10% of men are addicted to sex, pornography, etc. Among the impotent and liars, 10% say they don't struggle at all. Of course nowadays they may have some other sexual orientation. We can conclude therefore that 80% of men struggle with sexual temptation – meaning a total of 90% men struggle.

Acknowledging that we're in a war for our souls and striving to maintain our sexual purity is half the battle. Together we can successfully wage the war and be victorious. None of us are as strong as all of us. Less of me and more of we. The first banana to get pealed is the one that gets separated from the bunch. Faith is a fact and an act, the difference is in the doing. There is nothing wrong with struggling. It's when we give in that there is a problem.

Once you've made yourself accountable to somebody, you than must submit to their authority and expertise. Submission is often a most misunderstood concept. You cannot truly resist the devil, without having first submitted to God (Jas. 4:7).

Every electrical outage needs a voltage regulator. You can be powerful, but if you are not "harnessed" and regulated than you are not usable. You will only come out of bondage and come into your personal promised land as you are "harnessed" (Ex.13:18). Horses have bits and bridles. Though we are humans created in God's image, we too need to be bridled. It is our responsibility to yield and cooperate with God when He begins to harness and bridle us.

Submit to God, resist the devil, deny yourself, take up your cross and follow Jesus. (James 4:7; Matthew 16:24)

Remember the end of the wicked. (Ps.73:2-3,16-17) Remember God has better things for you both now and throughout eternity. (John 10:10; Mark 10:29-30) Eternity is a long time. How you live on earth will determine how you are known in heaven. Don't squander your life.

The Spirit gives Liberty

The Holy Spirit is "in and with" every child of God (John 14:17; II Corinth.13:14). You're not alone. Be led by the Holy Spirit as He forewarns you concerning temptation, the appearance of evil and potential dangers (John 16:13; Romans 8:14). Be prudent and foresee the evil the Spirit of the Lord shows you and ponder the path of your feet, lest you suddenly be removed and fall (Prov.22:3; 4:26). When the Lord shows you the way of escape, don't linger and flirt with evil but make a quick escape with haste and don't turn back to take a second look (I Corinth. 10:13). Rejoice knowing God has better things for you and that He'll reward you for your obedience (Hebrews 6:9; 11:6).

In 21 days (3 weeks) you can break any habit by perpetually defying it and replacing it with an alternative action and response. Defy the sin that seeks to destroy you! Rise up and go to war with it!

If you are married, remember that men cry for a release of testosterone approximately every 72 hours – 3 days. The first day after having had sex, your body may be more calm and cooperative. By day two business is picking up, that is your hormones are beginning to provide impulses. By day three not much else seems to matter as you've got to have it.

Nevertheless considering your wife's menstrual cycle, pregnancy, business travel and level of interest, you might need to practice self-restraint a bit longer. Ideally neither should withhold from the other in marriage. Unfortunately many do not always experience such generosity and attentiveness in marriage. It seems our culture has gotten to the point of practicing sex before marriage and then once married being bored with their partner. Undoubtedly this is a perverted and backward view and use of sex.

It's interesting to note that Jesus rose on the 3rd day. One song we used to sing in church says: "Let the glory of the Lord rise among us. Oh, let it rise!" The patriarch Abraham must have written that song when he, nearly being 100 years old, thought to be intimate with Sarah prior to the promised son Isaac who was to be born.

A satisfied man, both spiritually and sexually, is a happy and productive man. If you hit a homerun in the bedroom, you probably will also do better in the boardroom. Being fulfilled sexually can serve to stabilize your heart and mind providing more focus for work and productivity.

Ultimately fulfillment comes from delighting in your Creator, governing your bodily appetites, co-creating your world with divinity and serving humanity. Intimacy with God is paramount to manifest self-control in your sexuality. Disciplining yourself to be self-controlled will greatly enhance your life and make you whole.

Self Control – prophetic principles

The sex drive is not evil and therefore should not be ignored. It must be understood and controlled. What is evil is when you allow your body to take over the affairs of your life and essentially rule you.

It behooves us to evaluate and examine our urges to see whether they are of the flesh or the Spirit. Stimulation unaccounted for and blindly followed can be extremely dangerous. Merely going by feeling can be harmful.

Never put a question mark where God has put a period. No wed, no bed.

Life without an awakened spirit is purposeless and self-centered.

Godliness with contentment is great gain (1 Tim.6:6).

Many of us know WHAT we should be doing, but do not KNOW HOW. The will is present, but HOW TO PERFORM we don't know.

What we continually behold, good or bad, we are compelled to become.

There are many tempting parking spots on the road to success.

Feed the spirit and starve the flesh.

Thoughts produce images. Images lead to actions; actions form habits; habits lead to strongholds. (II Corinthians 10:3-6)

God intended for you by the strength of the spirit within to govern your flesh. Intimacy with God is paramount to manifest self-control in your sexuality.

Masturbation is not God's plan for man. It is essentially like playing tennis by yourself, not so fun.

When a person masturbates they set up that image in their mind as an idol and bow down to it.

You can be dead right as far as the world is concerned *but dead wrong* and committing sin as God sees it.

Self-control is the exercise of restraint over one's own impulses, emotions, and desires. Self control is exercised more easily when you have built a strong inner man through prayer and reading of God's Word.

It's your responsibility to control your body and mind. (Romans 12:1-2)

Evaluate and examine your urges to see whether they are of the flesh or the Spirit. Stimulation unaccounted for and blindly followed can be extremely dangerous.

Merely going by feelings can be harmful. A frog can give you a feeling and then urinate on you.

Accountability precedes recovery.

You cannot truly resist the devil, without having first submitted to God (James 4:7).

You will only come out of bondage and come into your personal promised land as you are "harnessed" (Ex.13:18).

How you live on earth will determine how you are known in heaven.

God has better things for you and will always reward you for your obedience.

Defy and go to war with the sin that seeks to destroy you!

Ultimately fulfillment comes from delighting in your Creator, governing your bodily appetites, co-creating your world with divinity and serving humanity.

4. Relating to the Opposite Sex and Sin

The way we relate to the opposite sex has much to do with the erecting of proper boundaries. Once established and erected, many of the overtures that would seemingly come our way will be contained by reason of the relational perimeters we have initially set.

The Bible tells us that we are to regard the younger women as sisters and the older women as mothers. (I Timothy 5:2) This mindset and inner attitude can be a moral guideline for internal valuations and categorizations of females we meet and with whom we interact.

Simply put, if you would not do that with your sister or mother, than you don't need to be thinking or doing that with any other lady. If you wouldn't lay hands on your sister and grope with her in the car, you should not be doing it with any other lady to whom you're not married.

Jesus said, If you have an urge to "Lay hands" on someone, do it on "the sick" (Mark 16:17). Tell Mr. Happy Hands to cool off and put his hands in his pockets. If you don't plan on marrying someone, you don't need to be getting involved in a relationship with them. God doesn't want you partaking of another man's wife or daughter. (Exodus 20:17) Don't covet a man's daughter or wife either as this prolonged enamoring of the mind could lead to the pursuit of a wrongful relationship.

Assessing Manhood

Having sex doesn't make you a man. Dogs can have sex. Manhood is determined by your ability to control your bodily appetites and rightly direct them according to God's will for your life.

Love is not lust. Love gives. Lust is insatiably selfish and only takes. Love is never in a hurry. Lust wants immediate gratification. Love is understanding and patient. Lust is not tolerant, demanding, and impatient.

Love is friendship set on fire. That means a friendship and relationship of trust must first be established prior to the exchange of words of love. Words apart from a commitment is meaningless. Talk is cheap, as is a fast thrill in the car's backseat. Ladies should never give the milk away for free if they want the man to buy the cow.

Adam, God's number one man, was placed in a blissful garden with a beautiful wife of his own. He had sweet fellowship daily with God, along with all his heart could desire. His manhood was established in that he was whole spiritually, socially, and sexually.

Yet when he sinned, a curse and painful toil took over his life (Gen.3:17-19).

Banished from the garden where God had originally placed him, Adam undoubtedly was sorrowful (v. 23). His act of disobedience however had been committed and the just recompense underway.

Cain, Adam's son, killed his brother Abel (Gen.4:9-10). The result of Cain's sin was poverty, the removal of God's peace, restlessness, and the life of a wandering vagabond (v.12). Such punishment was greater than Cain could bear, as his soul was overwhelmed with grief (v.13). Like his father Adam, Cain too was driven out of his personal promised land (v.14).

Both of these men, Adam and Cain, sought to assert their manhood but in the end wound up worst off than before. God had blessed, positioned and planted them, but they would not be content. Bent on rebellion they opened the door of disobedience to allow the curse to come in and devour them.

These two men show us that true manhood is found in submission to God and His purposes. Self-assertion is unnecessary as long as one is submitted to Almighty God and obediently following Him. Taking up your cross and denying yourself is the greatest display of manhood you could ever render before the eyes of God.

Sin continually crouches at the door to have us, but we must master it (Gen.4:7). We must never forget that sin takes you further than you want to go, keep you longer than you want to stay, and costs you more than you want to pay. Manhood is realized when you deny yourself, submit to God, and master sin.

Excessive sexual sin is often linked to inner hurts and troublesome wounds within the soul. Some of the inner attitudes and tendencies causing pollution are: pride, insecurity, lust, and restlessness. Manhood's development begins when self-awareness is realized and the transformation process has begun. Personal transformation must be desired and sought after.

**Relating to the Opposite Sex and Sin –
prophetic principles**

Nowadays couples have the honeymoon first: If it's a success, they have the engagement, and if that works out all right, they may have a wedding.

If you don't plan on marrying someone, you don't need to be getting involved in a relationship with them.

Words apart from a commitment is meaningless.

Sin is like eating cotton candy. Though it does not nourish you, it tastes good for a little while. The more you over indulge and eat eventually the sicker you'll feel.

Having sex doesn't make you a man. Dogs can have sex. Manhood is determined by your ability to control your bodily appetites and rightly direct them according to God's will for your life.

True manhood is found in submission to God and His purposes.

Love is not lust. Love gives. Lust is insatiably selfish and only takes. Love is never in a hurry. Lust wants immediate gratification.

Love is friendship set on fire.

Sin takes you further than you want to go, keep you longer than you want to stay, and costs you more than you want to pay.

Jesus said, "Sin no more, lest a worse thing comes upon you" (John 5:14). To avoid fornication God lets every man have his own wife.

Beware of optical adultery. Make a covenant with your eyes.

Know what God has portioned and allotted to you in this season. Be content therewith.

Everything is beautiful in its proper season. God is not saying NO, just maybe not NOW.

Love is understanding and patient. Lust is not tolerant, demanding, and impatient.

5. Destroying Delilah and Jezebel

Love righteousness and HATE iniquity (Hebrews 1:9). You cannot be nice and toy with temptation. You cannot flirt and play with a seductress. Samson tried and he lost everything! He lost his position in God as he went from being a mighty deliverer to a slave of the Philistines. He got his eyeballs plucked out, his hair cut off, and his dignity stripped from him. He became the town mockery.

Sinful tendencies and internal play with wrongdoing is deadly. Predetermine to say, "NO!" and shut the door on the devil in your life (Ephesians 4:27; Genesis 4:7).

Tell your flesh to shut up and obey. If your flesh continues to be defiant and resists you, fast and discipline it. Fasting spanks your flesh and shows it who is boss – the spirit man.

Devilish Delilah pressed Samson daily "with her words, and urged him, so that his soul was vexed unto death" (Judg.16:16). Delilah was on a mission to afflict and bind Samson (v.6). She would not rest until she stole his strength (v.15).

This is why God exhorts us not to give our strength unto women (Prov.31:3). The essence of all addiction is the addict's experience of powerlessness over a compulsive behavior, resulting in their lives becoming unmanageable. The addict is out of control. Sexual preoccupation takes up tremendous amounts of energy.

One young man once said, "Sex is like crack. It's like a drug. You've just got to have it. Then when you seek it out to get it, upon getting what you were after, you realize it's not all that it's made up to be. Yet you just had to have it."

Samson thought he could play with Delilah and still have his dynamite God-given power. Yet when Samson sought to shake himself to bring forth the divine strength needed to break free, he found that the Spirit of the Lord had quietly left him (Judg.16:20).

Jesus warned the church at Thyatira to not give place or permission to the false prophetess Jezebel. Jezebel was a self-proclaimed prophetess, teaching God's servants to commit fornication. She also taught them to eat food sacrificed to idols. Jezebel was seducing God's servants (Rev.2:20). Jesus said Jezebel and they who commit adultery with her will suffer tribulation (v.22).

Maybe Delilah and Jezebel have been making sport of you (Judges 16:27). You don't have to go down in defeat. Rise up and fight! Call out to the Lord for restoration and new strength. (Judg.16:28). Take the walls of lust and perversion down and come free into glorious and perfect liberty in Christ.

Be a man of God! Endure temptation and receive the blessing. "Blessed is the MAN that endures temptation: for when he is tried, he shall receive the crown of life, which the Lord has promised to them that love Him. Let no MAN say that when he is tempted, I am tempted of God: for God cannot be tempted with evil, neither does He tempt any man: But every man is tempted, when he is drawn away of his own lust, and enticed. Then when lust has conceived, it brings forth sin: and sin, when it is finished, brings forth death" (James 1:12-15).

Christianity is a strong man's religion. Anybody can yield to temptation and give into the seduction of sin. It takes a real man to walk alone and defy the works of darkness. Are you man enough to take up your cross and daily deny yourself to be all that you can be in God's army? Before you can conquer the world you must first conquer yourself! Your flesh is your biggest enemy.

Destroying Delilah and Jezebel –

prophetic principles

You cannot be nice and toy with temptation.

Every man is tempted, when he is drawn away of his own lust, and enticed. Then when lust has conceived, it brings forth sin:

and sin, when it is finished, brings forth death" (James 1:12-15).

Sinful tendencies and internal play with wrongdoing is deadly. Predetermine to say, "NO!" and shut the door on the devil in your life (Ephesians 4:27; Genesis 4:7). Tell your flesh to shut up and obey.

The eyes of a man are never satisfied, neither is hell. Don't go there!

Looking to the left and the right will only take you to hell beneath. Lift up your eyes, look up and think on that which is above.

What you continually look at gets bigger.

What we continually behold, good or bad,

we are compelled to become.

The mind generates and produces mental

images according to the thoughts, concepts

and ideas you give it to work with.

Flirt and play with a seductress and like

Samson you too can lose everything.

The essence of all addiction is the addict's

experience of powerlessness over a

compulsive behavior, resulting in their lives

becoming unmanageable.

The Holy Spirit is "in and with" every child of God. You're not alone.

Be led by the Holy Spirit as He forewarns you concerning temptation, the appearance of evil and potential dangers. Be prudent and foresee the evil the Spirit of the Lord shows you and ponder the path of your feet, lest you suddenly be removed and fall.

When the Lord shows you the way of escape, don't linger and flirt with evil but make a quick escape with haste and don't turn back to take a second look.

Before you can conquer the world you must first conquer yourself! Your flesh is your biggest enemy.

6. Deliverance from Demonic Influences

Every devil has an art. God does not want us to be ignorant of the devil's devices and strategies, which he uses to assault and destroy us (II Corinth.2:11). Below are some of the spirits related to sexuality and the body which we must war against to maintain our personal freedom.

spirit of infirmity (Luke 13:11) – "And, behold, there was a woman which had a spirit of infirmity eighteen years, and was bowed together, and could in no way lift up herself."

unclean spirit (Mark 1:23) – "And there was in their synagogue a man with an unclean spirit; and he cried out."

seducing spirit (1Tim.4:1) – "Now the Spirit speaks expressly, that in the latter times some shall depart from the faith, giving heed to seducing spirits, and doctrines of devils."

spirit of perversion (Isa.19:14) – "The Lord has mingled a perverse spirit in the midst thereof: and they have caused Egypt to err in every work thereof, as a drunken man staggers in his vomit."

spirit of whoredom (Hos.4:12) – "A spirit of whoredom [prostitution] leads them astray; they are unfaithful to their God."

spirit of fear (2Tim.1:7) – "For God has not given us the spirit of fear; but of power, and of love, and of a sound mind."

lying spirit (2Chron.18:22) – "The Lord has put a lying spirit in the mouth of these prophets of yours. The Lord has decreed disaster for you."

Satanic Assaults on Your Sexuality

Let us take some time to break down the operations and maneuvers of each of these demon spirits. God's people perish because of lack of knowledge (Hos. 4:6). We need to know how to war. God by His Word and Spirit will teach us how to fight and accurately annihilate the enemy of our souls (Psalm 18:34). One of the resources I am using in this chapter is Dr. Henry Malone's *Shadow Boxing*. Do please refer to it for an exhaustive study on all root spirits. Here are the spirits that affect your sexuality.

The *spirit of infirmity* creeps into your life during times of laziness and unproductive behavior while you are laying around and mentally most susceptible. Such a spirit can subtly come upon you during prolonged seasons of rest and tell you "You're sick." If you don't realize and acknowledge it as an outside influence, you may assume ownership of it and create an identity of personal illness.

This spirit also may attack you during times of great productivity and accomplishment to slow you down and thwart your progression. Some of the symptoms of the spirit of infirmity are lingering disorders of the body, weakness, feebleness, cancer, female problems, fungus, fevers, allergies, sinus problems, high blood pressure, attacks on your femininity and masculinity, arthritis, heart disease, and diabetes.

An *unclean spirit* causes you to overlook your personal hygiene and disregard your daily upkeep on a physical level. This spirit will also affect the way you run your home and cause you to slack in regard to cleanliness and tidiness. Disorderliness is often attributed to such a spirit. In its full blown manifestation, such a spirit will even cause you to delve into grotesque things such as playing with your food and misuse of your body. MTV's show *I Bet You Will* and the famous *Fear Factor* though humorous, are platforms for unclean and vile behavior that play on college kids need for cash.

A *seducing spirit* is a roving imposter that misleads and deceives. Girls who are called a "tease" are precisely that. They are cooperating with a seducing spirit to lead guys on and perhaps just for the fun of it, never intending to commit to a man. Others who get online via the internet and play as if they are somebody they're not and get members of the opposite sex all worked up for nothing are being used by a seducing spirit to mislead and deceive.

Another form of this spirit's deception is it paints a romantic picture, similar to soap operas, that an affair or loose sexual behavior is fun and fulfilling, when in reality it proves to be destructive in the end. Notice in soap operas you never see the stars brushing their teeth, washing their dirty clothes, changing the baby's diaper, or cleaning the house. Such shows are misleading and very much play on women's emotions and ability to fantasize.

A *spirit of perversion* makes a complete mess of you. It minimizes and reduces your level of concentration on important tasks, always wanting to divert you into some perverse pleasure. This perverse spirit will distort the true purpose of things and cause you to have a perverted view about life which short circuits you from properly relating to people and thereby gives birth to instability in your life.

Since such a spirit runs with the spirit of pride and a lying spirit (demons are like dogs and run in packs), acknowledging that you have a problem and need help is never an issue as these spirits will tell you, "You don't have a problem."

The spirit of perversion thwarts your productivity in everything you put your hand to, causing you to err and go astray. It literally hinders your focus and consistently derails you toward perverse sexual activity until it ultimately leaves you lying in your own filth and degradation, as a drunken man in his vomit.

Some of the outwardly visible manifestations of *a perverse spirit* are: homosexuality, bi-sexuality, multi-partner sex orgies, sadomasochism, unreasonableness, error (often in religious doctrines promoting loose sexual behavior), abnormal crankiness. Unreasonableness and abnormal crankiness are a big part of the spirit of perversion, as it will drive you until it gets to act out its fantasy through the aid of your physical body. It will settle for nothing less than its desire regardless of your daily priorities and wishes.

A *spirit of whoredom* seemingly is a deeper and more deadly sexually oriented spirit than even the perverse spirit, as it is essentially a spirit that causes you to fully commit yourself (body and soul) to fulfilling every form of lust. As people give themselves over to a sexual orbit and outlook upon life, everything being about sex, they basically wed this spirit of whoredom. It is then women often begin to sell their bodies for sex - harlotry.

Once you've walked the plank so to say with this spirit, it will take you into more heinous sex acts such as adultery, molestation, rape, and incest. At its inception however it may seem harmless. Yet it is vying for a closer proximity to your home and heart. Some of the ways it gains a closer proximity to you and continual abode with you is via pornography and masturbation.

Don't Be Afraid – Lie With Me Baby

A *spirit of fear* as it relates to sexual behavior will often make you go introverted and withdraw from social activities as thoughts of insecurity and shame overwhelm you. It will make you want to hide from whatever it is you have done that you are ashamed of. Conversely, the spirit of fear can also cause you to erroneously believe that if you do not have sex with a person that they will not like you and therefore discontinue dating you. Fear of loss will often compel young women to have premarital sex with someone they worry about losing.

The truth is if he'll leave you because you won't have sex with him, he's a loser anyhow and worth leaving. Before you can have a new beginning you first must have an old ending and rid yourself of people with mixed motives who don't have your genuine interest at heart.

Other manifestations of *the spirit of fear* in relation to one's sexuality are: torment, fright, nightmares, fear of death, faithlessness, lack of trust, paranoia, inferiority, inadequacy, shyness, rejection, worry, anxiety, critical spirit, tensions, stress, fear of failure, performance, fear of others opinions of you, migraine headaches, schizophrenia, insanity, phobias, sense of abandonment, fear of pain, fear of men or women, and fear of authority.

Women often fear rape which can cause fright and nightmares. Fear of losing somebody you're in a relationship with can cause torment. Feeling inadequate and inferior cause faithlessness as one doesn't believe in oneself and therefore doesn't expect others to want to be with them for any extended period of time. A spirit of fear can cause one to be critical of others in an effort to diminish others confidence so as to bring others down to their level of self-worth.

A *spirit of fear* often drives one to be performance oriented and thereby concentrate on what they *do* to make up for *who* they are or are not. If past relationships have gone sour and feelings of abandonment linger, it is quite possible for a person to lack trust toward the gender that hurt them. Mistrust can even grow into a fear of the opposite sex. Such a distorted view develops when one throws the blanket of generality over a whole gender. These kind of distorted views open the door for the spirit of perversion to come in and whisper how good it is being a homosexual or lesbian. Distrust toward a gender can cause you to fear authority figures of that gender. It is no wonder with all of the dysfunctions caused by the spirit of fear that God says, "fear has torment" (1Jn.4:18).

Lies are the devil's forte as he is the father of lies (John 8:44). A *lying spirit* likes to get in on the action as it pertains to your sexuality and bombard you with lies as to your looks. "You're ugly. Nobody likes you. You're too white. You're too black. You're too brown. You're hair color is messed up. You're too thin. You're too fat. You look just like your mother." The list goes on. God however says we are wonderful in our appearance as we were made in his image (Genesis 1:26-27; Psalm 139:13-18).

A *lying spirit* can sometimes work on you the moment you walk into a room full of other people and you begin to hear: "You're a tramp. You're not welcome here. Nobody wants you, you little whore. All the guys no about you." Or, if you're a guy, "You ain't gonna get any of these girls attention. They like so and so. You're not with it. How you gonna get a girl to look at you when you…. Everybody knows ______ about you."

In regard to committing sexual sin, a *lying spirit* will work overtime on you saying stuff like this: "Go ahead and do that. It's o.k. God understands. You need a release. Your wife's got a headache. She's not meeting your needs. You're not hurting anybody. Go ahead. This is the Lord speaking. Don't be afraid. I still love you. Besides last time you were in church not one brother greeted or acknowledged you. Church folks are all hypocrites anyhow! Go ahead and have fun! It's your life!"

Another method or avenue of attack for the lying spirit could be as follows: "Come on, everybody's doing it. David had several wives and concubines and he was a man after God's own heart. Go ahead. You love God. God will forgive you. After all He created you like this. Everybody's doing it. Even so and so is doing it and he's a deacon. Come on, let's get dirty!"

The truth however is wrong is wrong even if everybody is doing it and right is right if nobody is doing it.

One Life – One Wife

God has given man one life and the opportunity to marry one wife. Anything beyond this is deception.

Yet the spirit that dwells in us lusts…(James 4:5). You therefore must continually take up your cross and deny yourself.

Sometimes you don't need a demon removed from you, as much as you need something renewed in you – that is in your mind. (Romans 12:1-2) Be aware and know your own particular set of temptations and their peculiarities. Obtain from the Holy Spirit your battle plan and route of escape for such temptations prior to facing them on the frontlines of battle.

Foresee the evil snares which you will face once you walk out of the door and leave your house. "A prudent man foresees evil and hides himself" (Prov.22:3). Don't flirt with and entertain such temptations. Get built up in God and your identity in Christ so feelings of insecurity won't be resident within your soul. Feelings of insecurity can soulishly lead you to give into sin when another woman begins to look at you a certain way and tell you how wonderful you are. Make sure you and your spouse daily exchange words of affirmation and build one another up continually. The devil will come at any hour when you least expect it. Be on guard always never taking anything or anyone for granted!

Premeditate your route and means of escape. Predetermine your course of action prior to facing your enemy. Be prepared for the devil to entice you and push all the right buttons in an attempt to seduce you. Make a wholehearted commitment and know your weaknesses and potential pitfalls in advance.

Guard against the common traps that befall you and cause you to sin. Get a firewall and popup blocker for your computer. Drive another way to work if necessary. Have your secretary screen your phone calls. Take every necessary precaution. Inform your spouse of various temptations and Satan plots to snare your soul.

Gifts are given, but they must also be guarded and guided. Daily count your spouse a blessing and thank God for her or him. If you are single, thank God for the gift of being single and the grace to remain focused on Christ and the building of His kingdom.

3 Roots of Sexual Impurity

1.) Tiredness and Routine – Daily monotony can often cause you to be present in body and absent in mind. Countless people go to work daily and their heart is nowhere to be found in what they do. This is not a good thing. Nevertheless, such is reality. Lip service can commonly be given in the absence of any heartfelt affection or sincerity (Matt.15:7-8). We do well in the midst of routine to remember that we will be rewarded if we don't faint (Gal.6:9). Scripture repeatedly exhorts us to not be weary in well doing (2 Thes.3:13).

Men are hunters & fishers. Pursuing something whether it be a woman, a fish, a deer, or a business deal tends to be our nature. Men therefore should let God wire and program them to pursue Him and His heavenly calling for their lives. We all have a need for "newness" and freshness. Thankfully, God can provide us with both "newness of life" and "fresh oil" daily to assure us variety and spontaneity (Rom.6:4; Psalm 92:10). Our Lord makes all things new (Rev.21:5). The living God wants to give us richly all things to enjoy and daily load us with benefits (1 Tim.6:17; Ps.68:19).

Among the many "things" He wants to give us continually are new experiences, new and improved relationships and take us to new places. What a wonderful God we serve! All He asks of us is to remain full of faith and to be faithful to Him. Be full of faith for the fresh and new things God has in store for you and remain eternally expectant!

2.) Boredom – Idle time is the devil's playground. The idle soul shall suffer hunger (Prov.19:15). David, the man after God's own heart, became idle at the time he should have been in battle (II Sam.11:1-2).

The end result of his sabbatical so to say was adultery, murderer, and a stillborn child. Divine timing and being mindful of spiritual purposes is paramount to avoid distractions elsewhere. When you are possessed with heavenly vision and the God given mandate upon your life, the zeal of the Lord consumes you. Yet if you have shrunk back in your heart due to an evil heart of unbelief and thereby recoiled from your forward press toward your divine destiny, you can rest assured Satan will lull you to sleep with a lullaby. During such times of being inwardly down and out the devil will entice you to get up and out with the pleasures of sin. When all you can do is mope and be the devil's dope, you had better go and sit underneath the prophetic preaching of an anointed minister who can stir you afresh in your faith and divine purpose. Otherwise, you'll wind up laying around, purposelessly playing with your belly button, and letting the devil be your pimp.

3.) The Lust of the Eyes and flesh, combined with a Carnal, Unrenewed Mind – Jesus said the primary gate through which lust is conceived is the visual gate called the eyes

(Matthew 5:28). Notice Jesus never mentioned a woman looking and lusting. Apparently, men are more visually stimulated than women. Inward infatuation of the heart leads to inner adultery long before you every commit the act. God is concerned with the inner imagery of our heart and mind (Ezekiel 8:12). Only the Holy Spirit can delete your mental files and clean the chambers of your imagery. It is the spirit of holiness that gives heavenly vision. Evil thoughts result in evil manifesting in and around us. The only way to be delivered from evil is to accept God, His Word and hearken steadfastly unto Him (Jeremiah 6:19). A mind is a terrible thing to waste. Eyesight without insight will lead you to destruction. Hearken to the Word of the Lord and make haste!

Deliverance from Demonic Influences – prophetic principles

Before you can resist the devil, you must first submit to God.

There are many tempting parking spots on the road to success.

Starve your eyes from feasting on female flesh. Bounce your eyes away and increase your spiritual strength today.

Feed your spirit and starving the flesh will become easier as you develop a hunger for spiritual things.

A mind is a terrible thing to waste, misuse and neglect. For us to be whole in our soul, we must strive to fully develop our mind.

Sexual fantasies can leave you impotent relationally as they deceive and destroy your ability to embrace genuine intimacy – leaving you always present in body but absent in mind.

Masturbation is not God's plan for man. It is essentially like playing tennis by yourself - not so fun.

Sinful tendencies and internal play with wrongdoing is deadly. Predetermine to say, "NO!" and shut the door on the devil in your life.

Tell your flesh to shut up and obey. If your flesh continues to be defiant and resists you, fast and discipline it.

When a person masturbates they set up that image in their mind as an idol and bow down to it.

The truth is if he'll leave you because you won't have sex with him, he's a loser anyhow and worth leaving.

Accountability gives birth to godly authority.

Once you walk the plank with demon spirits, entering into all kinds of lust, they will take you into more heinous and destructive sex acts intended to imprison you for life.

Mistrust can even grow into a fear of the opposite sex.

If you don't realize and acknowledge demon spirits as an outside influence, you may assume ownership of their messages and create a personal identity.

Demons are like dogs and run in packs.

The spirit of perversion thwarts your productivity in everything you put your hand to, causing you to err and go astray. It literally hinders your focus and consistently derails you toward perverse sexual activity until it ultimately leaves you lying in your own filth and degradation, as a drunken man in his vomit.

Lies are the devil's forte as he is the father of lies (John 8:44). A *lying spirit* likes to get in on the action as it pertains to your sexuality and bombard you with lies.

Wrong is wrong even if everybody is doing it and right is right if nobody is doing it.

Foresee the evil snares the devil has positioned to trap you and destroy your life. Predetermine how you will respond and preserve your life. "A prudent man foresees evil and hides himself" (Proverbs 22:3). Predetermine your route and means of escape beforehand.

Make sure you and your spouse daily exchange words of affirmation and build one another up continually.

Guard against the common traps that befall you and cause you to sin.

Daily count your spouse a blessing and thank God for her or him.

Men are hunters and fishers. Pursuing something whether it be a woman, a fish, a deer, or a business deal tends to be our nature. Men therefore should let God wire and program them to pursue Him and His heavenly calling for their lives.

Idle time is the devil's playground. The idle soul shall suffer hunger (Proverbs 19:15).

Divine timing and being mindful of spiritual purposes is paramount to avoid distractions elsewhere. When you are possessed with heavenly vision and the God given mandate upon your life, the zeal of the Lord consumes you.

Inward infatuation of the heart leads to inner adultery long before you every commit the act.

Only the Holy Spirit can delete your mental files and clean the chambers of your imagery.

Evil thoughts result in evil manifesting in and around us.

Eyesight without insight will lead you to destruction.

7. The Sword of the Lord

The Lord said to Joshua, "Sharpen the knives and circumcise again the children of Israel" (Joshua 5:2). God wanted some sharp utensils with which to do some cutting away of the flesh. Interestingly, God said "circumcise again" the children. Circumcision is a type and shadow of circumcision of the heart. It typifies the inner cleansing that occurs when the sword of the Spirit cuts away the filthiness of flesh and spirit from us (Jeremiah 4:4; 2Corinthians 7:1). We all must undergo the sword of the Lord.

Those who run from this process of circumcision will find themselves continually going around the mountain and repeating particular lessons that God would have them to learn. When you repeat patterns you perpetuate the pain therein that results from that habitual sinful tendency.

God took Elijah to Cherith, which is the cutting place, where He further separated him for his heavenly calling (1 Kings 17:3). We too must also lay on God's operating table and pass through God's laboratory, wherein He will run various experiments on us and see what is in our hearts.

True circumcision is of the heart, within the hidden man of the heart (Romans 2:28-29). Please don't go running to the kitchen to grab a knife. Fathers in Africa, typically Muslim, often circumcise their daughters – cutting away the clitoris to remove the pleasure of sex. Thankfully, God doesn't do such things. If God created it and put it there you don't have to get rid of it. You do however have to control it and keep it in its rightful place.

Circumcision of the heart is a continual process that occurs as we go through various phases of life and encounter new circumstances that expose what is within us. As the dross within your heart rises to the surface and reveals itself, be quick to repent and allow God's Holy Spirit to cut it away.

Wield the sword of the Lord through the power of His Spirit and boldly deal with yourself (Ephesians 6:17). Take up the two-edged sword of the Word and rid yourself of all impurity (Hebrews 4:12).

Remember you are never alone in this battle against the flesh and worldly lust, as the Spirit of the Lord is with and in you (John 14:17). Keep your Bible with you to feed and strengthen your spirit. Keep this book nearby as well if you have to as a continual reminder of the goal, the prize of the high call of God in Christ Jesus. Read and meditate continually on God's Word and these truths until they get inside of you. Joseph came out of the prison into the palace because he had taken ownership of God's Word and made it "his word" (Psalm 105:19). Make God's Word your word and possess it fully without wavering. By doing so, you will also begin to possess your soul.

Pass this book and material like it on to a friend in need. Live offensively! Start a help group for sex addicts at your work place, nearest church, or in your city. By helping deliver others from such bondage, you in turn are further preserving your own liberty. As you become a deliverer to others, you will raise up a mighty army to fight the fight of faith with you. None of us are as strong as all of us. Together we are undefeatable. Have a heart for others struggling in that which you have obtained victory over. Use wisdom when ministering to the opposite sex or people within the same sin which you came out of. Work in pairs, remembering Jesus sent His disciples out two by two (Luke 10:1).

Submit your life to a local Pastor who can keep you accountable and will commit to check up on you periodically when you least expect it. Be transparent and honest with such a leader as they work for your good and have your best interest at heart (Hebrews 13:17). Your interaction and sincere desire to change will be an encouragement to them.

I will conclude this book by giving you some practical ways to combat and overcome the flesh, the devil and the seductress.

1.) Be sober minded, ready in and out of season, for your adversary the devil seeks to devour you as a roaring lion waiting for the opportune time (1Peter 5:8; 2Timothy 4:2).

2.) Speak the Word out loud – "It is written" (Matthew 4:1-10)

3.) Meditate on God's Word (Joshua 1:8)

4.) See, envision, visualize the word of the Lord (Jeremiah 2:31; Acts 26:19)

5.) Be a doer of the Word (James 1:22)

6.) Don't flirt with sin or the appearance of evil. (1 Thessalonians 5:22)

7.) Guard your heart and ponder the path of your feet, allowing God to order your steps so as to avoid or at least reduce the number of temptations you face daily. (Proverbs 4:23,26; 7:8) Don't go "near" the seductress corner. Avoid it altogether.

8.) Say "No!" with authority to your flesh and misdirected "friends", speaking out loud with intensity without feeling shy, awkward or guilty – begin with yourself (Matthew 5:37). Say "No!" aggressively to yourself and your unruly flesh when necessary and appropriate. Be mean to yourself once and a while.

9.) Let God be true and every man a liar (Romans 3:4).

10.) Trust in the Spirit of the Lord within you and don't doubt His warnings (John 16:13; Romans 8:14; 1John 2:20).

11.) Discern between both good and evil (Heb.5:14; 1 Corinth. 2:11).

12.) Remain transparent and accountable to men of God – the devil works in darkness and secret (Eph.5:12; John 7:4). Be a tattletale on the devil.

13.) Receive from anointed ministry that preaches holiness, the Lordship of Christ and self-denial (Hos.4:9). Hot sermons give birth to hot hearts. A fly never lands on a hot stove.

14.)   Shut the doors in your life and home through which the flesh and devil enter [TV, radio, newspapers, magazines – Victoria Secret catalog, computer] (Eph.4:27; Gen.4:7).

15.)   Love your spouse full force – be aggressively affectionate (Matt.11:12). Don't delay in expressing love today. As the song goes, "You've got to tell her about it."

16.)   Talk about your spouse in the presence of others, bragging and making your love openly known. Express sexual contentment in your conversation (Heb.13:5). Make sinners jealous of what you've got (Romans 11:11). You've got a good thing at home so your mind doesn't have to roam.

17.)   Realize that many churchgoers who claim to be saved are not sanctified and therefore are sent by the devil [often unbeknownst to themselves] to distract and destroy you with fleshly lusts and perversions. (Prov.7:17-23) The adulteress paid her religious vows and brought peace offerings to church, then sought to cheat on her husband while he was away (v.14).

18.)   No wed – No bed. (Hebrews 13:4)

19.)   Unrestrained   sexual immorality leads to poverty. Remember a whore is a deep ditch. (Prov.23:27)   Many mighty men have been slain by seducing women and left impoverished (Prov.6:26). Habitual and unbridled lust will wipe you out if God doesn't judge you first (Genesis 6:6-7).

20.)   Emotional   and   soulish wounds are the result of sex outside of marriage.   (Prov.6:33)   The "precious inner life" will be mutilated, robbed and utterly destroyed (Prov.6:26). Sensitivity to the Lord will be severed as the flesh takes over.

21.) Reproach and dishonor occur as a result of "free sex" and unbridled lusts. HIV, STDs are not worth bragging about. (Prov.6:33)

22.) Hell is hot and death is drawing near. (Prov.5:5; 7:27; 9:18; 27:20)

23.) You can have more if you don't settle for less. A gift of God is a virtuous woman, whose price is far above rubies, who causes your heart to safely trust and blesses you in every area of your life leaving your soul fat and flourishing. (Prov.31)

24.) Consider your ways and count the cost of your actions (Haggai 1:5; Luke 14:28,33). Sin will take you further than you want to go; keep you longer than you want to stay; and cost you more than you're willing to pay. Sin is the blast that doesn't last.

25.) Temporary pleasure is not worth long-term pain. (2 Corinth.4:18).

26.) Flattery works ruin and sets you up to think more highly of yourself than you ought. Pride and vanity will separate you from God and take you down into the depths of sin. Maintain a strong self-image in Christ so that you are not so needy of female affirmation. (Prov.6:24; 26:28)

Please add your own recommendations to this strategic battle plan to combat sexual immorality. Develop your own sexual recovery plan tailor made to your unique and peculiar temptations. Send me a copy of it as I would like to review and add more helpful information to this first edition of *Stop Lusting and Start Living*.

Let somebody else know about your commitment to sexual purity so together you can hold one another accountable. Having a comrade to participate with in such a good work is encouraging and further fans the flames of enthusiasm for successful living. As you steadfastly strive for relational intimacy with the living God, sexual impurity will become a thing of the past.

Get ready! Your best days and your blessed are ahead of you!   Continually remind yourself of the great and precious price Jesus paid for you when He shed His own blood on Calvary's tree. He who Christ Jesus sets free is free indeed! The blood of Jesus can make the foulest clean. Now stand fast in the liberty wherewith Christ has set you free and don't be again entangled with the yoke of bondage (Galatians 5:1).

Christ's pain was your gain! His agony purchased your liberty. He endured Calvary so you could be free throughout eternity. He died for you. Will you now take up your cross and live for Him?

Pray with me now, saying:

"Jesus, I thank you for dying for me. You died on the cross naked and not ashamed. That is how I come to you today – naked and open. Yet I am ashamed of my sins. Jesus, it was my sins that crucified you to that tree. It was for my sins that you endured a brutal death. Forgive me Jesus. Cleanse me from my sins. Liberate me within. Come by the power of Your Holy Spirit and renew me. Create a clean heart within me. Send now Your Holy Spirit to change me and help me live for you. I surrender my life to you Jesus. From this day forward, I ask you to live big in me and make my life what it ought to be. In Jesus' Name. Amen."

The Sword of the Lord – prophetic principles

Inner cleansing occurs when the sword of the Spirit cuts away the filthiness of flesh and spirit from us.

When you repeat patterns you perpetuate the

pain therein.

True circumcision is of the heart and is a

continual process.

Make God's Word your word and possess it

fully without wavering. By doing so, you

will also begin to possess your soul.

By helping deliver others from bondage you

in turn are further preserving your own

liberty.

None of us are as strong as all of us.

Together we are undefeatable.

Hot sermons give birth to hot hearts. A fly never lands on a hot stove.

Christ's pain was your gain! His agony purchased your liberty. He endured Calvary so you could be free throughout eternity. He died for you. Will you now take up your cross and live for Him?

Never put a question mark where God has put a period.

God will render unto you the fruit of your thoughts. Be extremely careful therefore what you allow to circulate and camp out in your mind.

Thoughts produce images. Images lead to actions; actions form habits; habits lead to strongholds. Do your thoughts amount to a pile of feces or an indestructible fortress?

Personal transformation must be desired and sought after.

Present your body to God as a living sacrifice and be renewed in the spirit of your mind. It's your responsibility to control your body and mind.

Life affords us ample opportunity to be offended with people, but love enables us to endure all things.

You can be dead right as far as the world is concerned *but dead wrong* and committing sin as God sees it.

Faith is a fact and an act, the difference is in the doing.

It is your responsibility to yield and cooperate with God when He begins to harness and bridle you.

Anticipate demonic attack. Premeditate your route and means of escape. Predetermine your course of action prior to facing fleshly lusts and the enemy of your soul.

8. Mended for Marriage

Make Jesus your all in all. He alone will sustain you daily. Don't put unrealistic expectations on people. We all live in flesh and blood. Therefore we are all prone to frailties and inappropriate behavior. Keep your eyes on Jesus Christ, not the Christians of Christ. We are all hypocrites in some sense of the word as in some area of our lives we are not yet perfected. In other words God is still working on all of us. Be gracious to all therefore knowing that you too are in need of mercy and grace.

Ministry must begin with you. Learn to minister to yourself. Develop the greatest love of all, that being for you. Perhaps you are torn or broken within due to some unexpected relational disappointment or relational trauma you experienced. As painful as it was, you cannot change it by continually thinking about it.

Get over it therefore for your own sake! Stop renting out space in your mind to the person who wronged you! Forgive and let live! Forgive yourself if necessary.

If you went through a divorce, take those pictures of your former spouse and get rid of them! Trash or burn them. Get rid of the old so God can bring in the new! You cannot have a new beginning without first having an old ending. Have a funeral service if need be with some intimate friends and family who can support you as you grieve over the loss of that someone who was once dear to you.

Be crucified with Christ afresh so thereafter you can walk in newness of life (Galatians 2:20; Romans 6:4). Die to your past so you can live unto your future. Get your foot out of yesterday and put it into today! Be fully and joyfully present no longer mourning about yesterday. Be resilient and take what life gives you as an adventure and surprise!

Your butt is behind you and your eyes are in front of you! Therefore if someone leaves you, say "Next!" and move on! As harsh as it may seem it is very needful for the sanity of your mind and the stability of your spirit. All things work together for good when you love God (Romans 8:28). Therefore rejoice as your Creator can create a new life story for you and that far better than the past!!!

Here are some things to do for yourself immediately.

A.)Take time for personal repairs.

Some times we need our souls to be restored. God promises to restore and strengthen our souls (Psalm 23:3; 138:3). Jesus found the disciples "mending their nets" as they had been torn (Matthew 4:21). Our souls often are in need of repair due to past hurts and wounds we're holding on to

(Luke 4:18). Allow Jesus to heal your broken heart.

B.)Forgive those who have wronged and disappointed you.

If you cannot forgive, your heavenly Father cannot forgive you (Matt.18:34-35). You may not *feel* like forgiving the person who you have ought against, but you can do so by faith and release them unto God. Cast your cares, even those who have been uncaring toward you, on the Lord as He cares for you (1Pet.5:7). Only God can turn a person's heart around anyhow. The king's heart is in the hand of the Lord and like a river He can turn it wherever He wants it to go (Prov.21:1). Maybe God is allowing that person to test your heart to see what is in you. Stop trying to play God and strive for purity yourself. When you get out of the way and give place to God, He can begin to work (Rom.12:19). Don't avenge yourself, but rather give place to God's wrath as vengeance belongs to Him. His is a righteous judge and will surely judge the living and the dead. You however should sow mercy as you too might need some in your hour of need (Matt.5:7).

C.)Repent for not walking in love.

If you would be brutally honest with yourself, you could admit that you have used others to gratify your fleshly lusts and not truly walked in love toward them. Love gives as it does not seek its own. Lust however is quick to take and get for itself. Walking in love requires a conscience effort daily. Lust simply takes and comes quite natural to most of us. Love gives and that grinds against our inbred selfishness.

Repent for placing unrealistic expectations on people, including your family members and spouse. Again, true love does not make such demands. True love seeks to serve others at your own expense (1Corinthians 13). Repent for not being sensitive to the needs and feelings of others. People that are most close to us are the ones we most often neglect. Sad it is but true. People have emotional and physical needs that need to be attended to. Such needs cannot merely be met just to get the job done without the willingness of heart that soothes and settles the soul.

D.)Remove walls and stereotypes built in your mind toward the opposite sex.

Bad sexual experiences and unkind words scar. Once you've been healed, purpose in your heart to love again and be vulnerable to your spouse who God has given you. If you're single, determine that you will not categorize the opposite sex and make vague categorizations which pigeon-hole people. Blanket statements tend to suffocate you and keep you from entering into meaningful relationship due to erroneous stereotyping.

E.)Shut the door on the devil and forbid him access.

Build yourself up in the Word and prayer so as to build an impenetrable fortress in your inner man. God exhorts us to give no place to the devil (Eph. 4:27). If you're giving place to the devil, don't get mad at God when the curse begins to devour your life. When you have dinner with a thief, don't look surprised when your wallet is missing afterward. The devil and his demon spirits within his "bag of tricks" are thieves, sent from hell to devour and destroy your life (Jn.10:10).

We can cleanse our way by giving close heed to God's Word and walking circumspectly in the light of it (Psalm 119:9;

Eph.5:15). Daily discipline yourself to hide God's Word in your heart (Colossians 3:16). Meditate upon God's Word day and night. Speak it to yourself and the situations you face throughout the day. Be a doer of the Word and you shall experience great success and full prosperity (Josh.1:8).

Sanctified and Satisfied Singles

Singles rejoice in the gift of being single. It's truly a wonderful season of your life not to be hurried through or despised. Don't wish away your years. Maximize each and every season of your life for the glory of God. Being single has many pluses, the least of which are:

1. You have nobody to bump into in the middle of the night.

2. You have nobody to answer to at home (apart from God) once you've reached adulthood.

3. You can attend to things without distraction.

4. You have less bills to pay.

5. You have less emotions to juggle and care for.

6. You have less complaints to hear.

7. You have more time on your hands to do that which you like.

8. You have fewer responsibilities.

9. You can patiently assess all of your options for matrimony without being in a hurry to commit to the wrong person.

10. You can travel without having to ask permission or buy an extra plane ticket.

11. You are more at liberty to spend time with your friends.

12. You can learn to cultivate joy and happiness within

Happiness must be cultivated and developed within. It does not come from without. Get joy and peace now while you're single. Then when it is time for you to marry, you won't be entering marriage empty, but rather happy and fulfilled already. That is you'll be bringing something to the table, rather than looking to take something. If you're not happy before marriage, you won't be happy after marriage. Happiness is a decision and it begins with you.

Don't stir up love before the time. Know the times and seasons of God for your life.

Rejoice in your present season and don't diminish the importance of it. Preparation time is not lost time. You don't find happiness in marriage. You must take happiness into marriage. In other words, you must be complete yourself before entering marriage.

Cultivating Contentment
and Making Marital Bliss

Married couples must rejoice with one another. Men are exhorted to rejoice with the wife of their youth (Prov.5:18). I guess the Bible has to tell some folks to rejoice and be happy as it doesn't come natural for everyone. God here is commanding us to rejoice! God says it twice. "Rejoice in the Lord always: and again I say rejoice!" (Phil.4:4). You do a double rejoice once in a while and you'll get a breakthrough in your marriage.

I told one young man to go home and begin jumping up and down with his wife on their bed and he'd get a spiritual breakthrough. They called me that night laughing like a bunch of little kids, full of joy and exuberance. Accessing the God kind of life isn't difficult. It's so simply attained most people miss it and let it pass them by.

Jesus wants your wife's breasts to always satisfy you (Prov.5:19). That means if your going to daydream about sex, it should be with your wife. If you're going to think about breasts, make sure it is your wife's. Be ravished always with her love. Be seized and taken away by her love. Rave and get goo-goo eyed about her love. Be overcome with joyous emotion and delight in her love. If you're not there yet ask Jesus to help you.

Pray with me now and say:

"Jesus, help me get carried away with my wife's (husband's) love. Cause ______ (your spouse's name) to get carried away with my love. Let us rave over one another. God cause us by Your Spirit to get wild and crazy about one another as when we first met and began our courtship. Jesus, You're the God of the resurrection, so please resurrect those feelings and that supernatural love within me and within us again."

Get captivated with your spouse again. Let your love begin to bubble up and overflow. If you have to, fake it before you make it. Call those things that are not as though they were (Rom.4:17). Prophesy to yourself and that spouse of yours. Say, "Honey, I tell you I just am so in love with you I'm beside myself. I can't stop thinking about you. You sure are a wonderful person. You've been so good to me. I thank God every time I think of you."

Somebody may think that's a lie. No, you're declaring that which you want to be. You can have whatsoever you say (Mark 11:23). You're just rightly applying the Scriptures to your relationship and circumstance. As you do God will confirm your word with signs following and do that which you speak in His ears (Num.14:28; Mark 16:20).

Get together again. Sit down and reflect. Meditate and ponder your marital history. Cherish the memories God has given you and call the good times to remembrance. Revival is nothing more than calling to remembrance that which God has done already for you. Do it and it won't be long before the Holy Spirit will be welling up on the inside of you and you'll be feeling like you ought to.

Creatively pursue love and romance with your spouse to keep your love relationship hot. Seek knowledge and godly instruction if necessary to help change your mindset toward your spouse. Put yourself around people and resources that will affirm your goals to revive and renew your marriage. Don't sit among the ungodly and expect some deep heavenly revelation about restoring your marriage. Go to the people of God, them who have it going on. You can't give what you don't have. Go to them who have a good marriage and value preserving it.

Some other books which might be good to read:

- 501 Practical Ways to Love Your Wife and Kids, by Roger Sonnenberg

- 501 Practical Ways to Love Your Husband and Kids, by Jennifer Baker

- Wild at Heart, by John Eldredge

- How to Make Love All the Time, by Barbara Deangelis

- The 5 Love Languages, by Gary Chapman

- Breakthrough for A Broken Heart, by Paul F. Davis

- Update Your Identity, by Paul F. Davis

Having a wide perspective and differing views about marriage can be very helpful. We all come from different backgrounds and ideological orbits based on our past upbringing and experiences. God exhorts us to dwell with our wives "according to knowledge" (1Pet.3:7). Apparently, the logical side of a man needs to be able to process all of that which is taking place within the female to whom he is wed.

Prayer is the next piece of advice given by God to help keep the union strong. The more we pray together, the more likely we are to stay together. This I know to be a truth as my ex-wife rarely if ever prayed with me. Prayer invites God to come into the marital union and interact with both parties. The Spirit of God can then begin to work positive changes within each person and further bring both together in marital harmony.

Sexual expression is often hindered for a woman if love and affection is not given throughout the day to build up to the time of intercourse. It's like a crock pot that takes time to simmer. Some of the ways you can express love toward one another prior to sexual intimacy are:

1. Giving gifts

2. Acts of service

3. Quality time

4. Physical touch

5. Words of affirmation

Next to a spiritual encounter with God Himself, a sexual encounter is probably the most remarkable experience any person can enjoy on this earth, because it involves every aspect of the physical self. It is more than the bringing together of sexual organs, more than sensual arousal of both partners, more even than mutual fulfillment in orgasm. It is the experience of sharing and self-abandon in the merging of two persons, expressed by the biblical phrase "to become one flesh" (Genesis 2:24). God created woman as a perfect "fit" to help man with his sexual drive. Man on the other hand was made in such a way by God to be able to secure and stabilize a woman's emotions while nurturing, assuring and comforting her.

Sex after marriage however is not always nirvana. When reality sets in after the honeymoon, many come to realize that sexual appetites differ. Women tend to not need sex as often as men. One Saturday night live episode portrayed this quite well. They had a few women breathing in disgust and saying, "I was happy at rest, but then he got all aroused when he started taking Viagra. Ugh, thanks Viagra."

Sometimes sex is like a half-court shot. It can be hit or miss if you don't invest the time and interest. Other times one gets more from it than the other. Just as a car with differing horse power and cylinders have to be driven different, so to do people with differing sex drives need to be handled emotionally and physically.

After you've done all you can do to improve your sex life, you have to simply leave it in God's hands. You don't want sex to become an idol, or like a god in your heart – as it is to so many. Keep sex in its proper perspective. Whether you're getting all your needs met or not, remember you are still accountable to God to maintain your purity of heart so you don't hinder your relationship with Him. "Kiss the Son, lest He be angry, and you perish along the way" (Ps.2:12). In all your getting of sex and developing of marital bliss, don't forget to give God a kiss and hold on to righteousness.

Mended for Marriage – prophetic principles

Be crucified with Christ afresh so thereafter you can walk in newness of life (Galatians 2:20; Romans 6:4). Die to your past so you can live unto your future.

All things work together for good when you love God (Romans 8:28).

When Adam was lonely, God created for him one wife, not ten friends.

No wed, no bed. If you're getting hot and bothered take a cold shower, go to the gym, call a brother in the Lord who you can pray with.

No good thing will God withhold from them that walk uprightly. Wait on the Lord and He will satisfy you fully spirit, soul and body.

Marriage was made in heaven and for the earth. Believe God and He will bless you in the fullness of time by bringing you into a perfect marital union with the person of His choosing for your life.

Eternity is a long time. How you live on earth will determine how you are known in heaven. Don't squander your life.

A satisfied man, both spiritually and sexually, is a happy and productive man. If you hit a homerun in the bedroom, you will have increased momentum to hit a homerun in the boardroom.

Author Contact

Paul F. Davis can be contacted for Counseling, Professional Speaking, Consulting, Coaching (professional & relational), Conflict Resolution and much more at the following below.

RevivingNations@yahoo.com

www.PaulFDavis.com

www.Linkedin.com/in/worldproperties

www.Facebook.com/speakers4inspiration

www.Twitter.com/PaulFDavis

Among 70+ books by Paul F. Davis

Breakthrough for a Broken Heart

Update Your Identity

Almighty Matchmaker

Are You Ready for True Love?

Healthy Relationships

Love Poems

Supernatural Fire

God versus Religion

A State of Emergency!

Waves of God

Back Cover

This book is a sword of deliverance and battle plan for sexual freedom.

Lust will take you further than you want to go, keep you longer than you want to stay and cost you more than you want to pay. Once ensnared it can be awfully difficult to break away.

What you do with your body effects your mind. The sex drive is not evil and therefore should not be ignored. It must however be understood and properly controlled.

You do not have to be a slave to your own lusts. Your body does not have to be your master. This book will show you how to:

- Get a grip on your flesh.

- Harness and possess your soul.

- Govern and rule over your bodily appetites.

- Avoid seduction and enticements.

- Discern the origins of urges and feelings before being drawn away by them.

- Differentiate between spirit, mind and body.

- Practice eye control on demand.

- Cultivate meaningful relationships.

- Fight to preserve your personal integrity.

- Live your life to the fullest.

- Put sex in its proper place.

- Properly evaluate and establish your manhood.

- Esteem women as God created them and see them more than sex objects.

- Know yourself and others by the Spirit.

- Live freely in the Spirit and cut the strings of seduction.

Promiscuous sex is like eating cotton candy. Though it does not nourish you, it tastes good for a little while. However the more you indulge and eat eventually the sicker you'll feel.

Having sex doesn't make you a man. Dogs can have sex. Manhood is determined by your ability to control your bodily appetites and rightly direct them according to your

life's purpose.

Love is not lust. Love gives. Lust is

insatiably selfish and only takes

Life is meant to be lived, not enslaved.

Liberation is yours for the taking. Stop

lusting and start living!

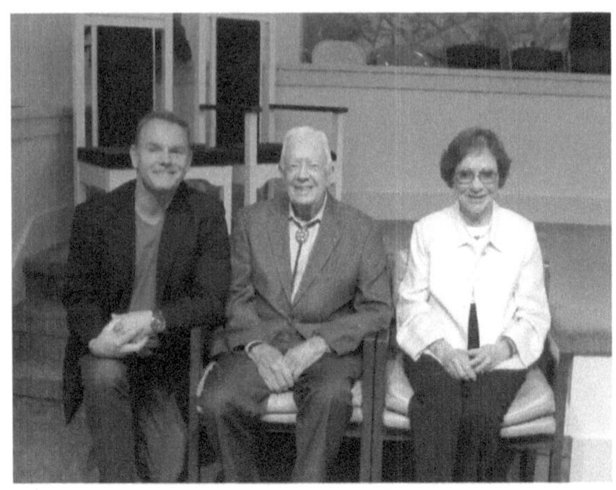

Paul with former United States President

Jimmy Carter and his wife Rosalynn

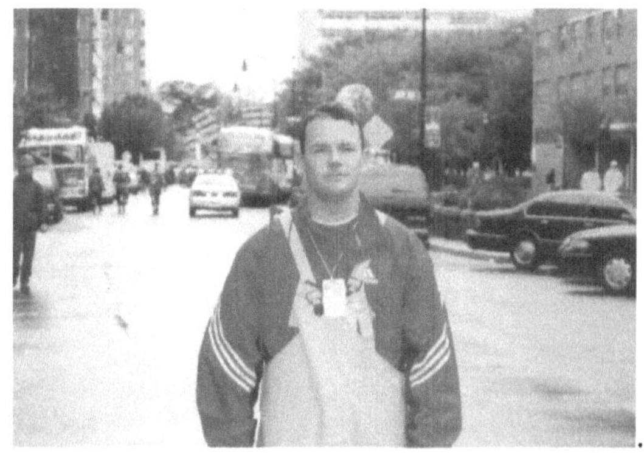

Paul in front of World Trade Center Tower 7, "Ground Zero" in New York City where the terrorist attack against the United States was committed on September 11, 2001.

Paul F. Davis is a Worldwide Minister, Motivational Speaker, Wellness Trainer, Life Coach and Author of 70+ Books who has touched 89 nations serving the U.S. Military, Companies, Cruise Lines, Churches, Schools, Colleges and Universities across the globe.

Paul provided rescue relief with the Salvation Army the first week of September 11th, 2001 at "ground zero" in New York City following the bombing of the World Trade Center. Paul traveled to Pakistan twice after 9/11, the nation where Paul believed Osama Bin Laden was hiding; prior to Presidents Bush and Obama pursuing and killing him therein.

Paul was raised by his grandfather, a U.S. Army retired Lt. Colonel. Paul's cousin is a retired U.S. Army Ranger and Paul's uncle served in the U.S. Navy. Paul has spoken on sexual assault & harassment prevention and suicide prevention for both the U.S. Army and Air Force. Paul served as an intern for the U.S. Embassy in Timor Leste when Hillary Clinton was the former Secretary of State.

Paul F. Davis is a Talent Development Trainer and Education Consultant who has served as a College & Career Counselor at Texas A&M International University and for the American China Exchange Society. Paul has earned 4 Master degrees with honors from New York University (Global Affairs), Michigan State College of Law (Global Food Law), the University of Alabama (Health), and University of Texas (Educational Leadership).

I pray God will be with and bless you!

I'd love to hear from you about how this book has blessed your life, your goals for the year, and how I can further help you.

Paul F. Davis

www.PaulFDavis.com
www.EducationPro.us
www.Linkedin.com/in/worldproperties
www.Twitter.com/PaulFDavis
RevivingNations@yahoo.com